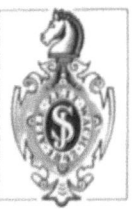

Magdalena Graf-Rüegg

Krebs Cancer

dennoch Hoffnung auf Leben   *A Second Flowering*

Springer-Verlag
Berlin Heidelberg New York
London Paris Tokyo
Hong Kong

Magdalena Graf-Rüegg
Böcklinstraße 9
CH-9000 St.Gallen

ISBN 978-3-540-50734-5   ISBN 978-3-642-45658-9 (eBook)
DOI 10.1007/978-3-642-45658-9

CIP-Titelaufnahme der Deutschen Bibliothek

Graf-Rüegg, Magdalena:
Krebs – dennoch Hoffnung auf Leben = Cancer – a second
flowering /
Magdalena Graf-Rüegg. – Berlin; Heidelberg; New York;
London; Paris; Tokyo; Hong Kong: Springer, 1989

Library of Congress Cataloging-in-Publication Data

Graf-Rüegg, Magdalena, 1936–
Krebs, dennoch Hoffnung auf Leben = Cancer, a second
flowering
Magdalena Graf-Rüegg.
        p.   cm. English and German. Bibliography: p.

1. Breast–Cancer–Psychological aspects. 2. Art therapy.
I. Title. II. Title: Cancer, a second flowering.
RC280.B8G69   1989   616.99'449'0019–dc19
89-31232

Gesamtherstellung: Appl, Wemding
2125/3114-543210 – Gedruckt auf säurefreiem Papier

2125/3114-543210 – Printed on acid-free paper

Krebs führt oft zum Tode

Aber es scheint Fälle zu geben, in denen die
Bedrohung durch Krebs den Beginn des Lebens
bedeutet.

Die Suche nach sich selbst, die Entdeckung des
Lebens, das zu leben dem innersten Bedürfnis ent-
spricht, kann eine der stärksten Waffen gegen die
Krankheit sein.

Cancer often kills

Yet there seem to be times when getting cancer can
become the beginning of living.

The search for one's own being, the discovery
of the life one needs to live, can be one of the
strongest weapons against disease.

Lawrence LeShan

Geleitwort

Der vorliegende kleine Kunstband mit Aquarellen von Frau Magdalena Graf-Rüegg und den kurzen Begleittexten spiegelt eine schwierige Lebensspanne wider. In dieser Zeit mußte sie erfahren und verarbeiten lernen, was es bedeutet, mitten im jungen, aktiven Leben von Brustkrebs betroffen zu sein. Niederschmetternd und bedrohlich nistete sich die unheilvolle Diagnose in ihr persönliches Dasein ein.

Neben Angst und Ungewißheit keimten indessen bald auch hoffnungsvolle Fragezeichen auf: Könnte diese Krankheit auch „Gutes" bringen? Kann neben Verzweiflung auch Hoffnung wachsen? Lohnt es sich zu kämpfen, statt zu resignieren?

Malerisch versuchte Magdalena Graf-Rüegg auszudrücken, wie sie den Beginn der Krankheit erlebte, wie sie die Operation und die nachfolgende längere chemotherapeutische Behandlung empfand und wie die anfängliche Trauer sachte einer Morgenröte wich. Nach neuer Persönlichkeitsfindung suchte sie neue Wege des Ausdrucks, die sie heute im Wissen, mit vertrauender Liebe gesegnet zu sein, weitergeht. Die Musik spielte für sie dabei eine unterstützende Rolle, und die (wiedergefundene) Malerei half ihr, Krankheit und Behandlung – trotz zwischenzeitlich erfolgtem Rückfall – positiv zu erleben und zu verarbeiten. Die letzten Bilder des Bandes strahlen denn auch Lebensfülle und Vertrauen aus:

Dank – Lob – Freude – Gott.

Frau Magdalena Graf-Rüegg lebt in St. Gallen, Schweiz. Sie wurde 1936 geboren, ist verheiratet mit einem ortsansässigen evangelischen Pfarrer und ist Mutter von vier erwachsenen Kindern. Nach der Ausbildung als Kindergärtnerin besuchte sie ein Jahr lang die Zeichenakademie in Tirlemont, Belgien. Mit 40 Jahren (1976) erkrankte sie. Nach der Brustoperation und nachfolgender unterstützender Chemotherapie begann sie – nach jahrelanger fami-

Foreword

The present slim volume of watercolours by Magdalena Graf-Rüegg and their accompanying brief texts, some of them written by herself, reflect one particular, difficult period of the artist's life: a time when she had to learn, and to learn to cope with, what it means when breast cancer strikes in the middle of a young and active existence. The appalling diagnosis lodged deep in her personal being, shattering, full of menace.

Soon, however, amidst the fear and uncertainty, hopeful questions began to stir as well. Could this illness also lead to something positive? Can hope grow up beside despair? Should she give in or fight?

In her paintings, Magdalena Graf-Rüegg tried to express her growing awareness of her illness, the experiences of surgery and the long chemotherapy which followed, and the way in which her initial grief slowly gave way to the light of dawn. Having found herself anew–in spite of cancer–she sought new avenues of expression, and lives today in the knowledge of being blessed by trust and love. Music accompanied this search, and the rediscovery of painting helped her to experience and cope with illness and treatment in a positive way, despite relapses. The last pictures in this book radiate fulfilment and trust:

thanks–praise–joy–God.

Born in 1936, Magdalena Graf-Rüegg lives in St. Gallen in Switzerland with her husband, a Protestant pastor, and four grown-up children. After training as a kindergarten teacher she studied at the Academy of Drawing in Tirlemont, Belgium, for a year. At the age of 40 she developed breast cancer. It was after the initial operation and subsequent supportive chemotherapy that she again took up lessons in music and painting, interrupted years before by the demands of her family and work. The disease set off a reawakening of the artistic gifts

liär und beruflich bedingter Unterbrechung – sich wieder dem Musik- und Malunterricht zu widmen. Die Krankheit wurde zum Anlaß, die im Alltag verschütteten künstlerischen Gaben und Bedürfnisse wieder zu aktivieren. Die vorliegende Bildserie entstand im Vorfeld der 3. Internationalen Konferenz über die Primärtherapie des Brustkrebses, an welcher über 500 Fachärzte aus 38 Ländern teilnahmen. Mit ihren 12 selbstkommentierten Aquarellen nahm Frau Magdalena Graf-Rüegg an der begleitenden Kunstausstellung des Kongresses teil und erregte durch die vertrauensvolle Schlichtheit und Wirklichkeitsnähe von Bild und Wort erhebliches Aufsehen.

Bilder und Texte dieses kleinen Bandes bereichern und ermutigen den Betrachter und Leser; inmitten von Krankheitsbedrohung und Ungewißheit läßt sich die Entdeckung machen, daß es ein erfülltes Weiterleben gibt. Wir hoffen, daß dieser Kunstband Betroffenen und Betreuern helfen möge, neue Kräfte für die Zukunft zu schöpfen.

St. Gallen, June 1988

and goals which had become buried in everyday life.

The present series of pictures came into being during preparations for the Third International Congress on Primary Therapy of Breast Cancer, which was attended by over 500 cancer specialists from 38 countries. These 12 watercolours, together with the artist's comments, were included in the art exhibition which accompanied the conference and were greatly admired for their trustful simplicity and the truth to reality of both words and pictures.

The pictures and texts in this little book will enrich and encourage the reader, showing, in the midst of the threat and insecurity of illness, that it is possible to recollect oneself and discover that a fulfilled life still awaits one–despite cancer. It is our hope that this collection will help all those who suffer from cancer and those who care for them to experience such supportive strength and–in spite of uncertainties–move hopefully forwards on their journey of discovery into the future.

Agnes Glaus
Hansjörg Senn

Dank

Thanks

Meiner Familie und meinen Freunden gegenüber er-
füllt mich tiefe Dankbarkeit für die entgegenge-
brachte Liebe und Geborgenheit.

Herrn Prof. Dr. med. Hansjörg Senn und Ober-
schwester Agnes Glaus danke ich besonders für die
ärztliche Betreuung und auch für ihren Einsatz, der
zum Entstehen dieses Bändchens beigetragen hat.

Ein spezieller Dank gebührt Alfred Kobel,
Kunstmaler, der mich im Zeichnen und Malen aus-
bildete und lehrte.

Donald Wipf, Musiker, möchte ich herzlich
danken für seine musikalischen Anregungen.

Herrn Dr. Fred Kurer danke ich für die Über-
setzung der Texte ins Englische.

I am filled with deep gratitude to my family and
friends for the love and security they give me.

I thank Prof. Dr. med. Hansjörg Senn and Ma-
tron Agnes Glaus particularly for their medical
care, and also for their part in bringing this book
about.

Special thanks are due to Alfred Kobel, artist,
who taught me drawing and painting.

Many thanks to Donald Wipf, musician, for his
musical encouragement.

Thanks to Dr. Fred Kurer for translating the
texts into English.

Magdalena Graf-Rüegg

Krank geworden

Fallen ill

Diagnose:
Mammakarzinom

Diagnosis:
Cancer of the breast

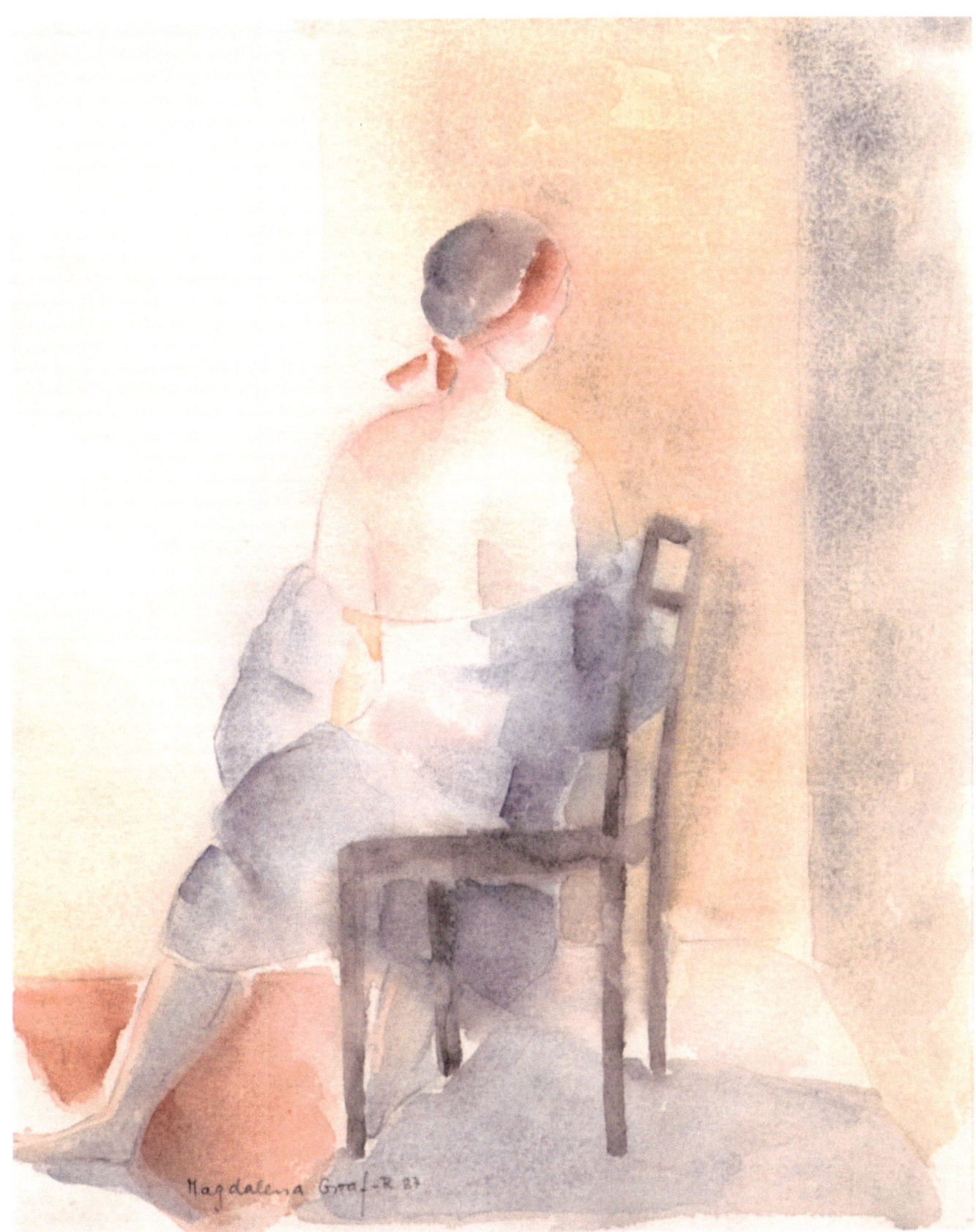

Magdalena Graf-R 23

Hoffnung
oder Verzweiflung?

Hope
or despair?

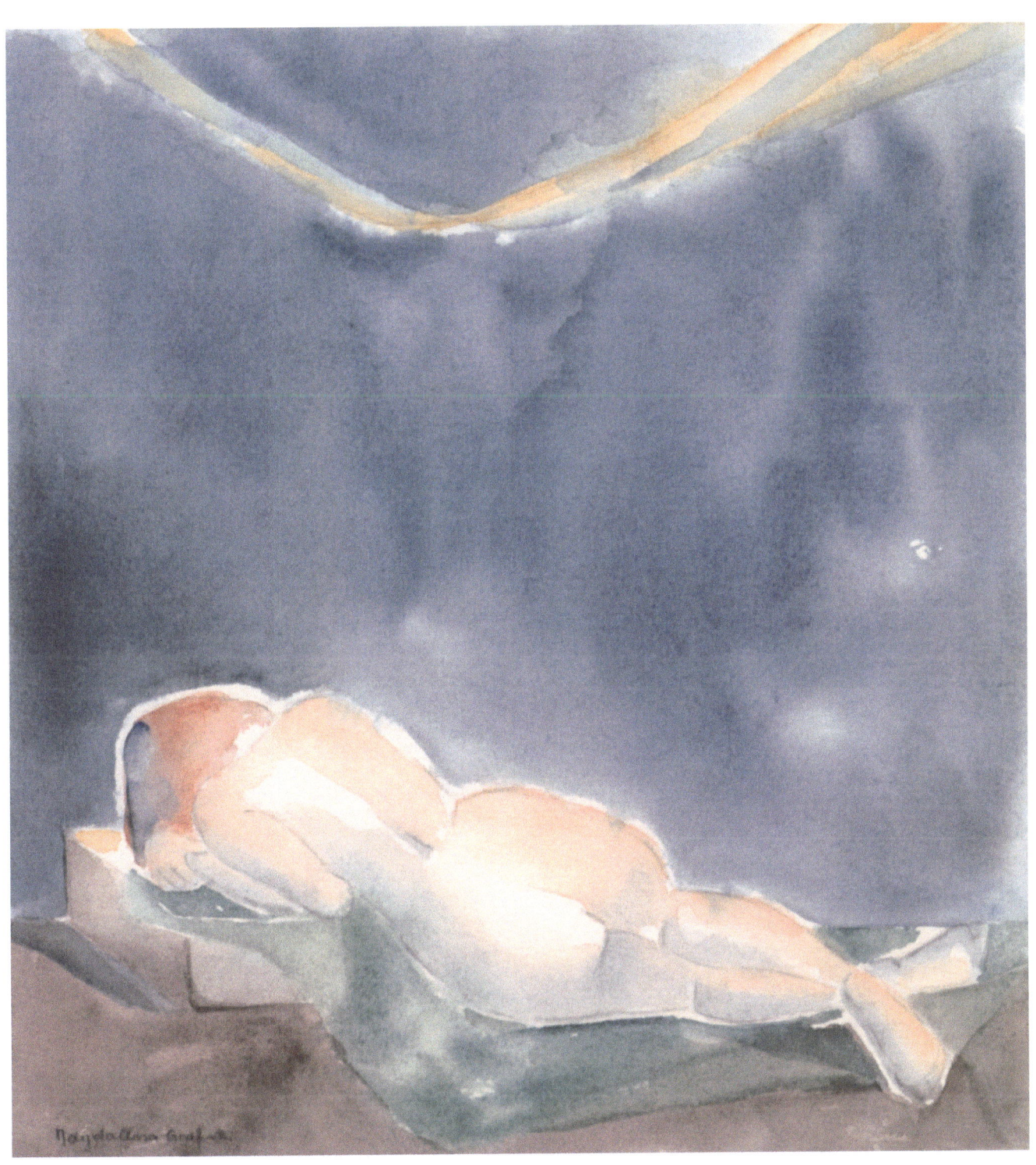

Resignation
oder Kampf?

Resignation
or fight?

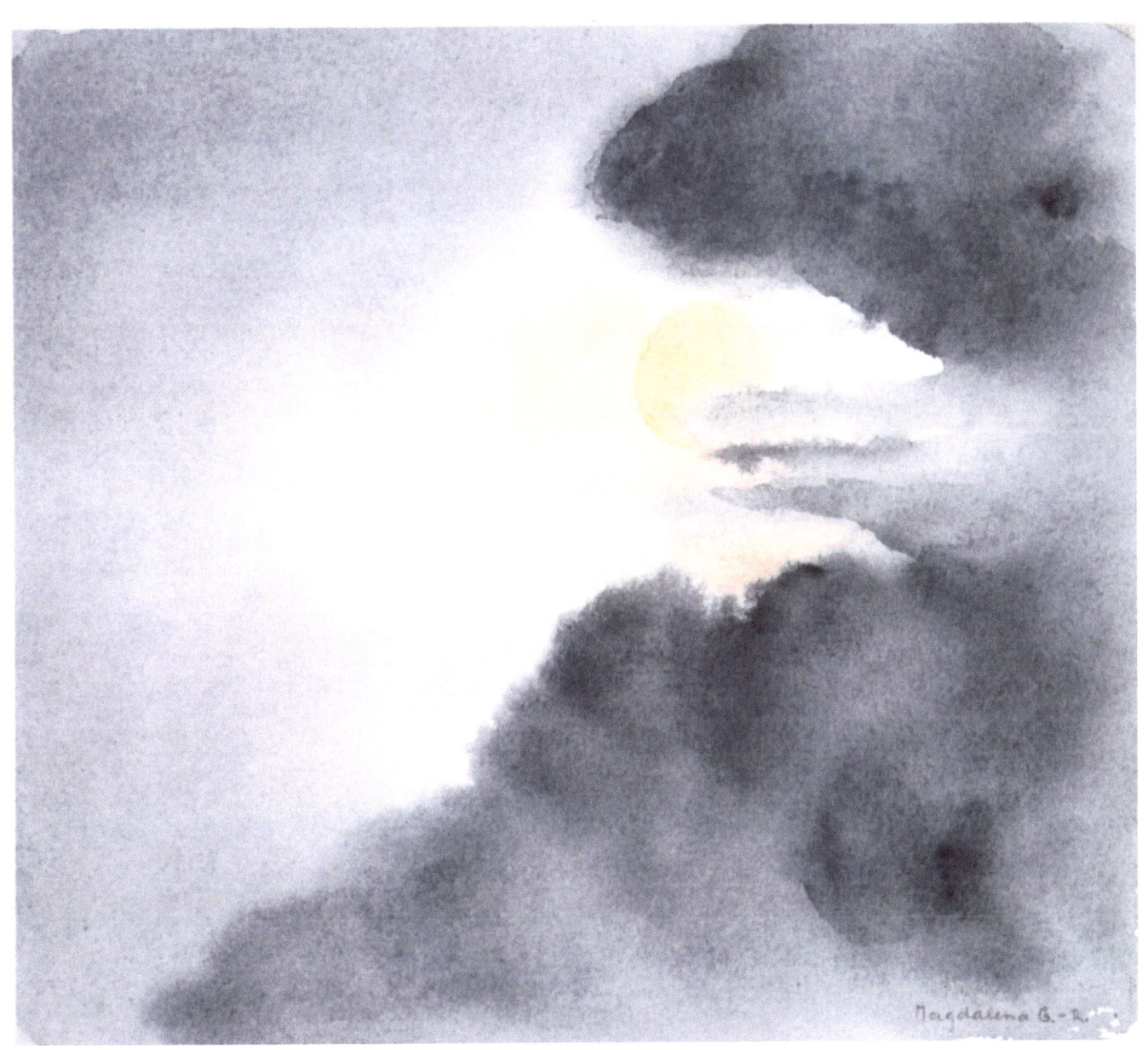

Chemotherapie   Chemotherapy

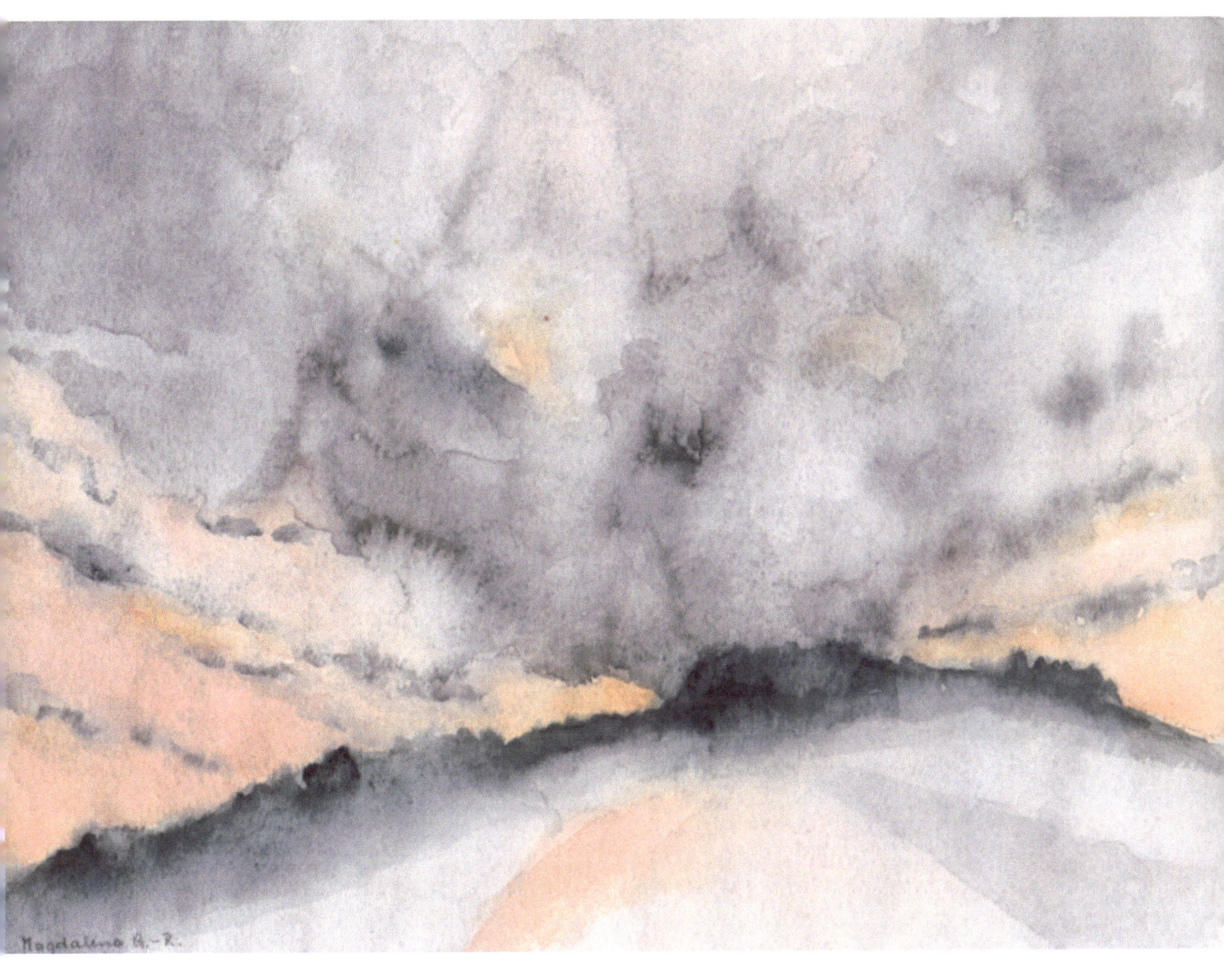

Magdalena H.-R.

Der Morgen
nimmt die Nacht
in den Arm

Morning
embraces night

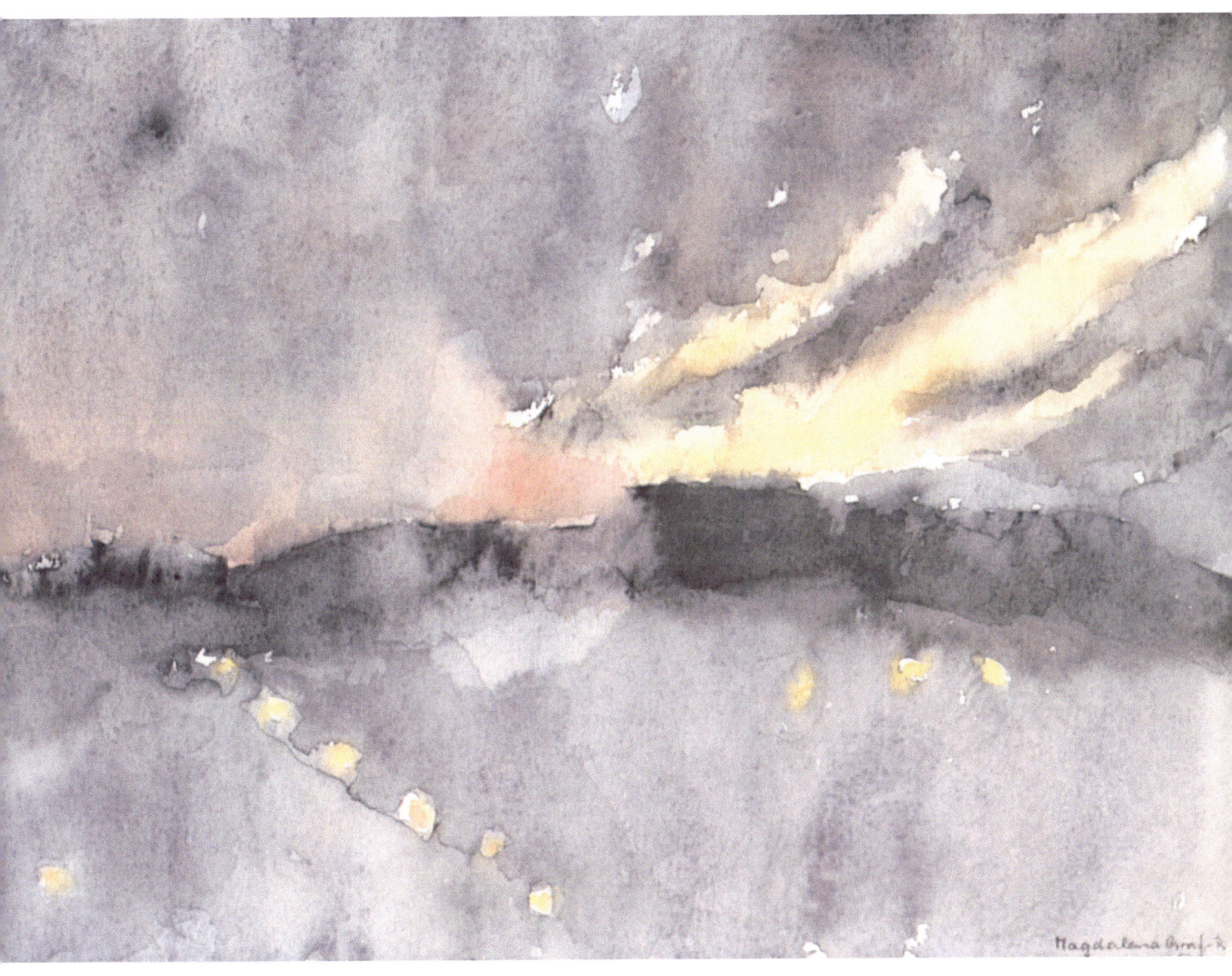

Magdalena Graf-R.

Neue Wege	New ways
suchen	looking for them,
finden	finding them,
gehen	going them

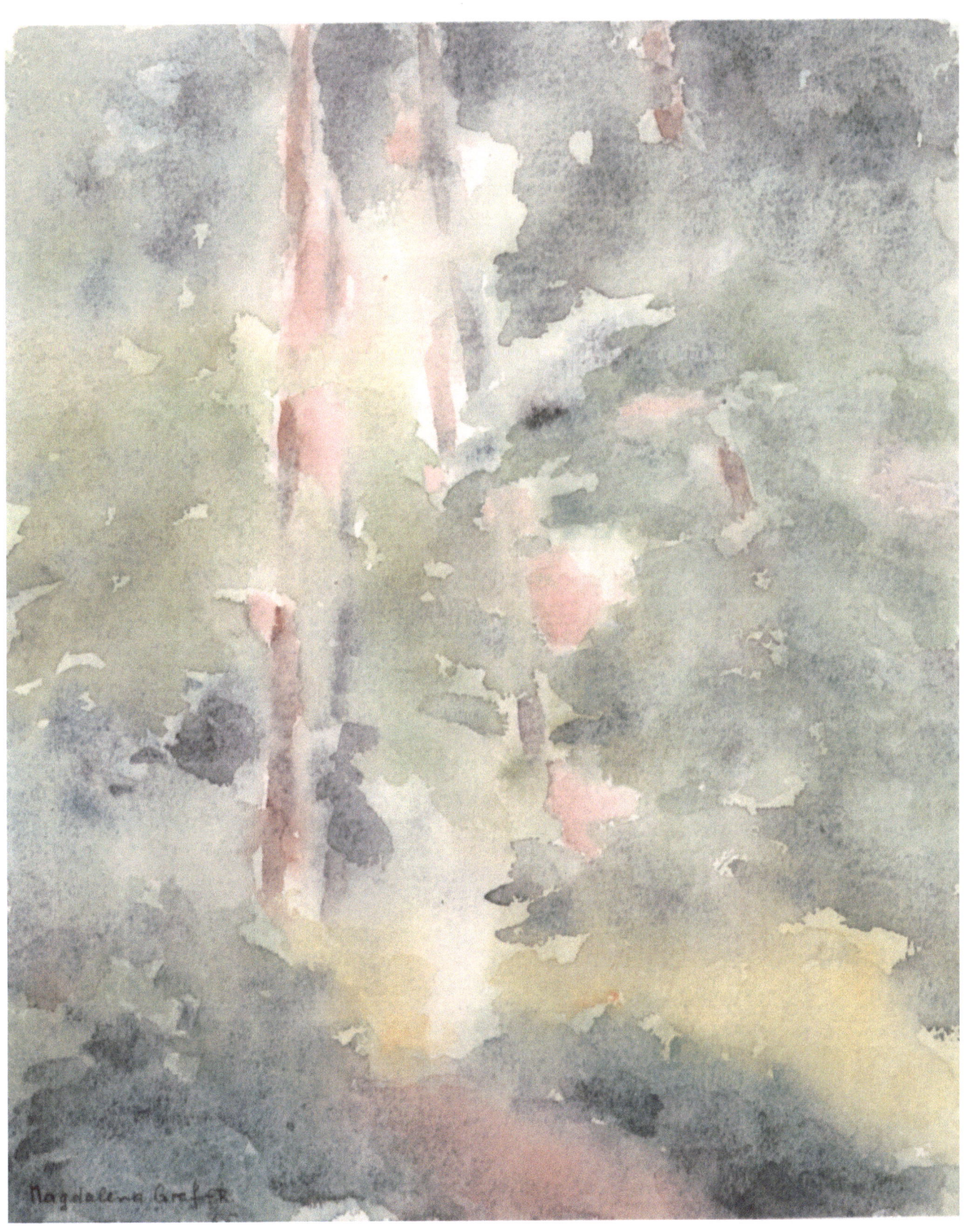

Magdalena Grafok

Liebendes Vertrauen
vertrauende Liebe

Loving trust
trusting love

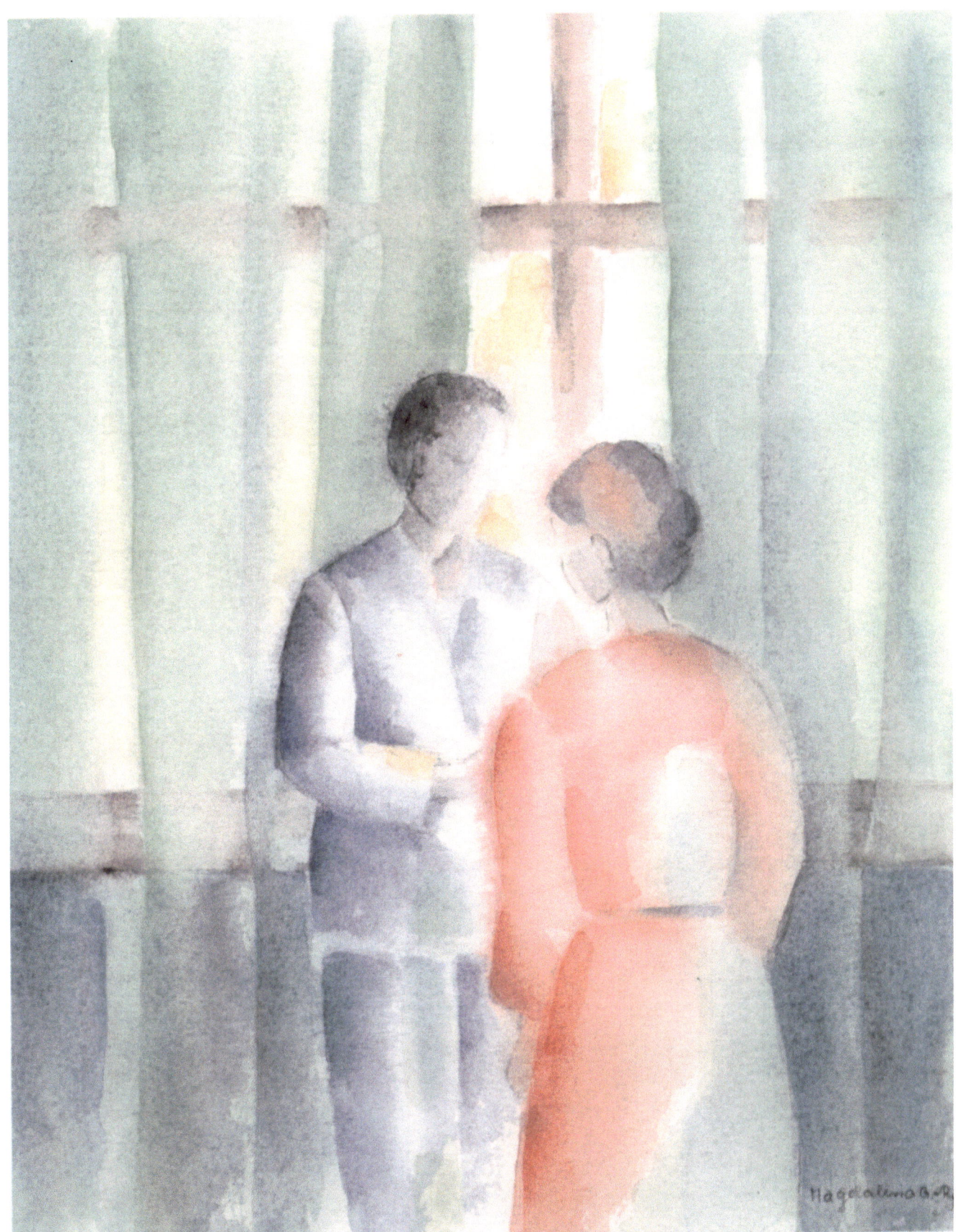

Musik

Das ist Musik:
sie befreit dich,
indem sie dich tiefer bindet.

Bernt von Heiseler

Music

This really is music:
by binding you
it sets you free.

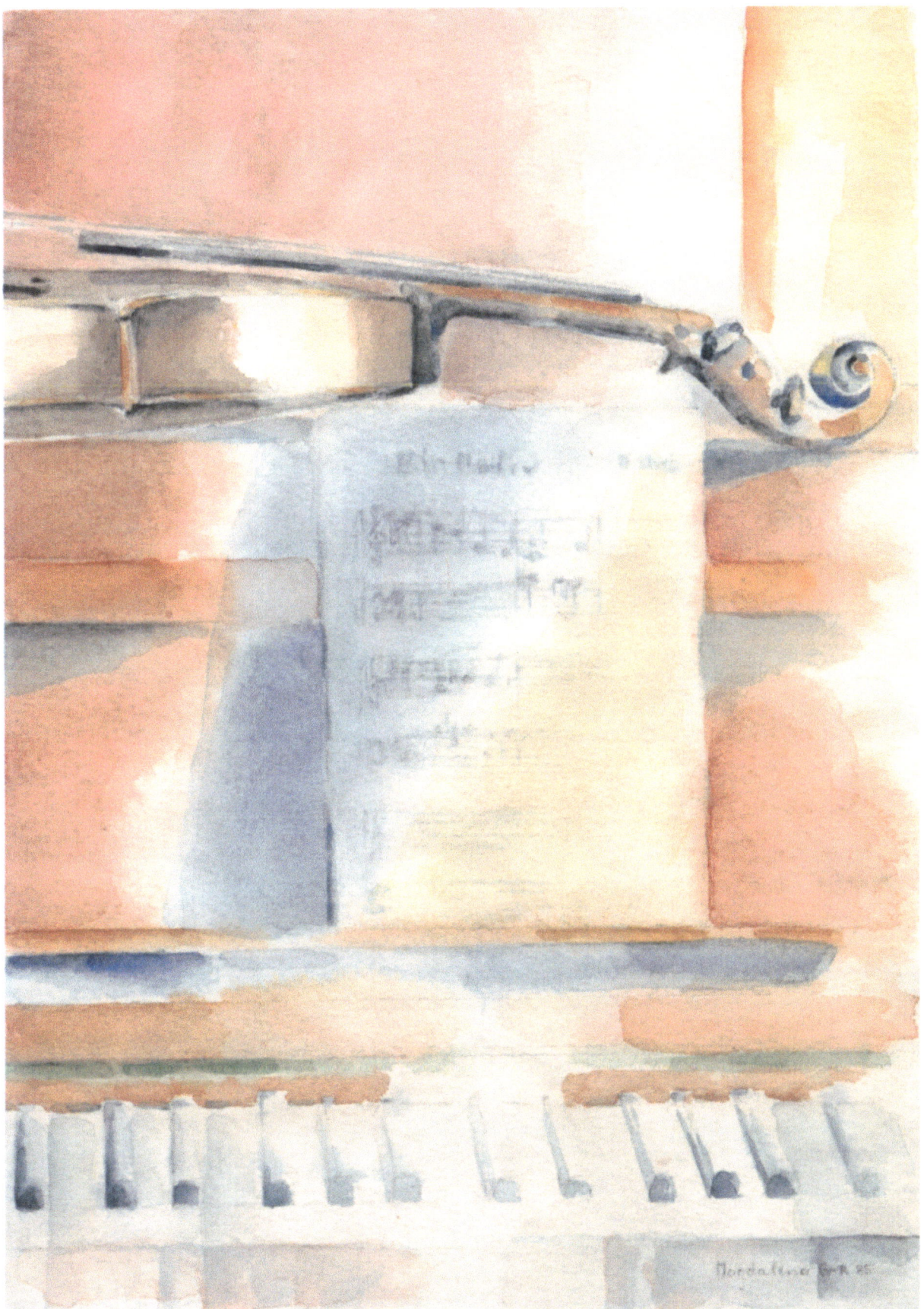

Malerei

Painting

Malerei und Farbe –
sind sie nicht von der Liebe inspiriert?
Ist die Malerei nicht allein
der Widerschein unseres inneren Selbst?

Isn't painting,
aren't the colours inspired by love?
Isn't each painting
a reflection of man's inner self?

Marc Chagall

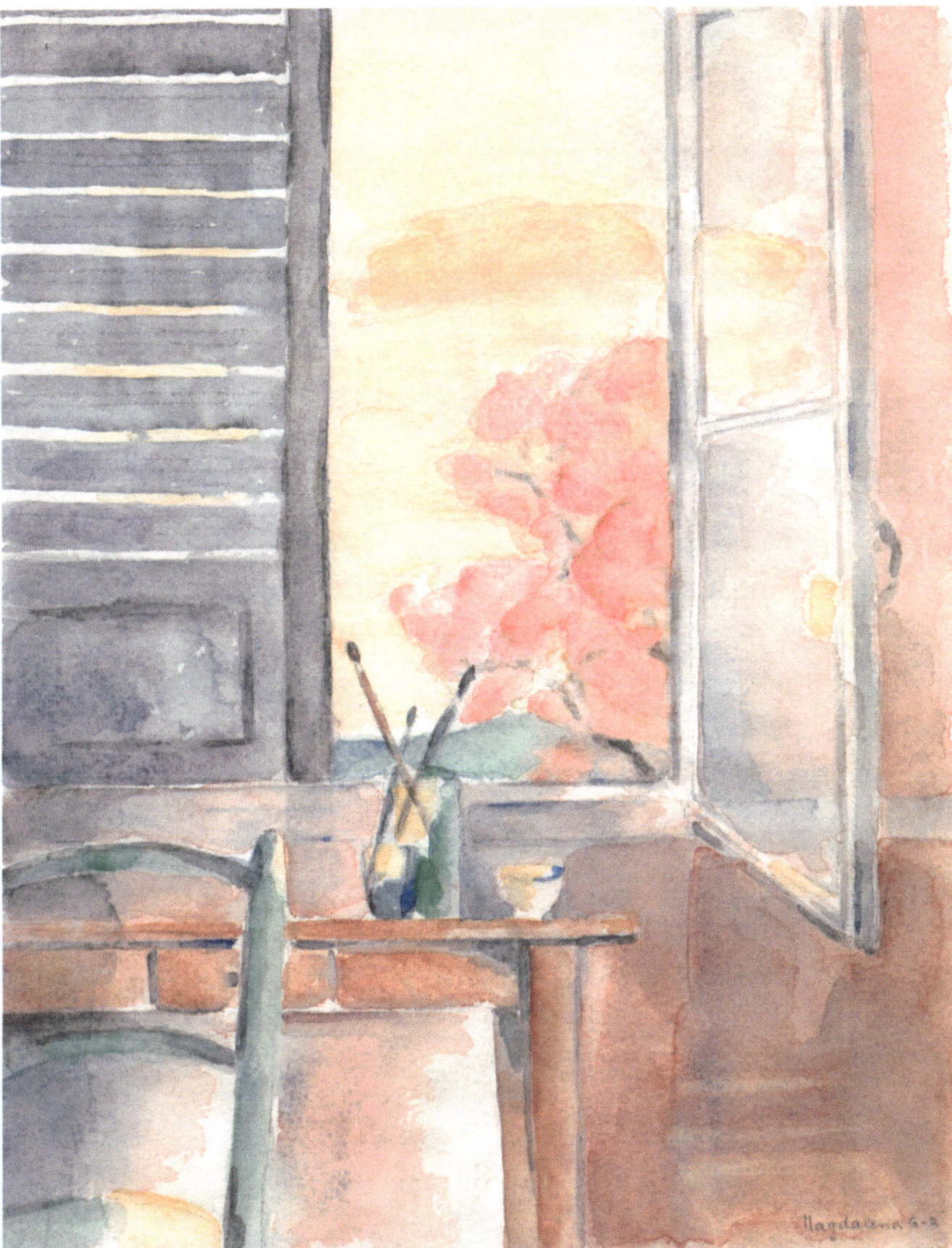

Der römische Brunnen

The Fountain in Rome

Auf steigt der Strahl und fallend gießt
er voll der Marmorschale Rund,
die sich verschleiernd überfließt
in einer zweiten Schale Grund;
die zweite gibt, sie wird zu reich,
der dritten wallend ihre Flut,
und jede nimmt und gibt zugleich
und strömt und ruht.

Up soars the jet and, falling, fills
The circle of the marble bowl,
Which, veiling itself, overspills
Into a second bowl below;
The second wells up, becomes too rich,
And floods the third with its excess,
And each one both receives and gives,
Both flows and rests.

Conrad Ferdinand Meyer

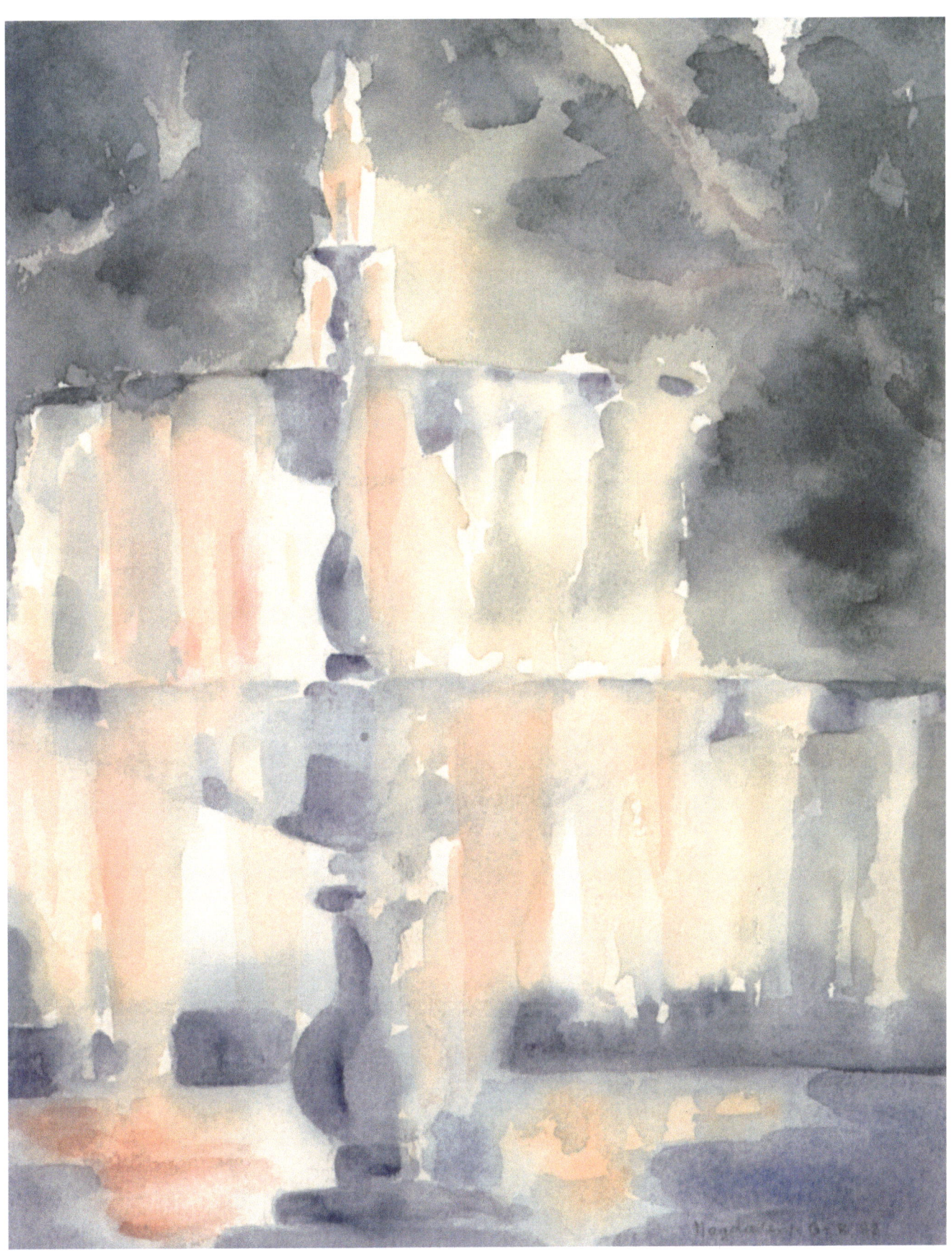

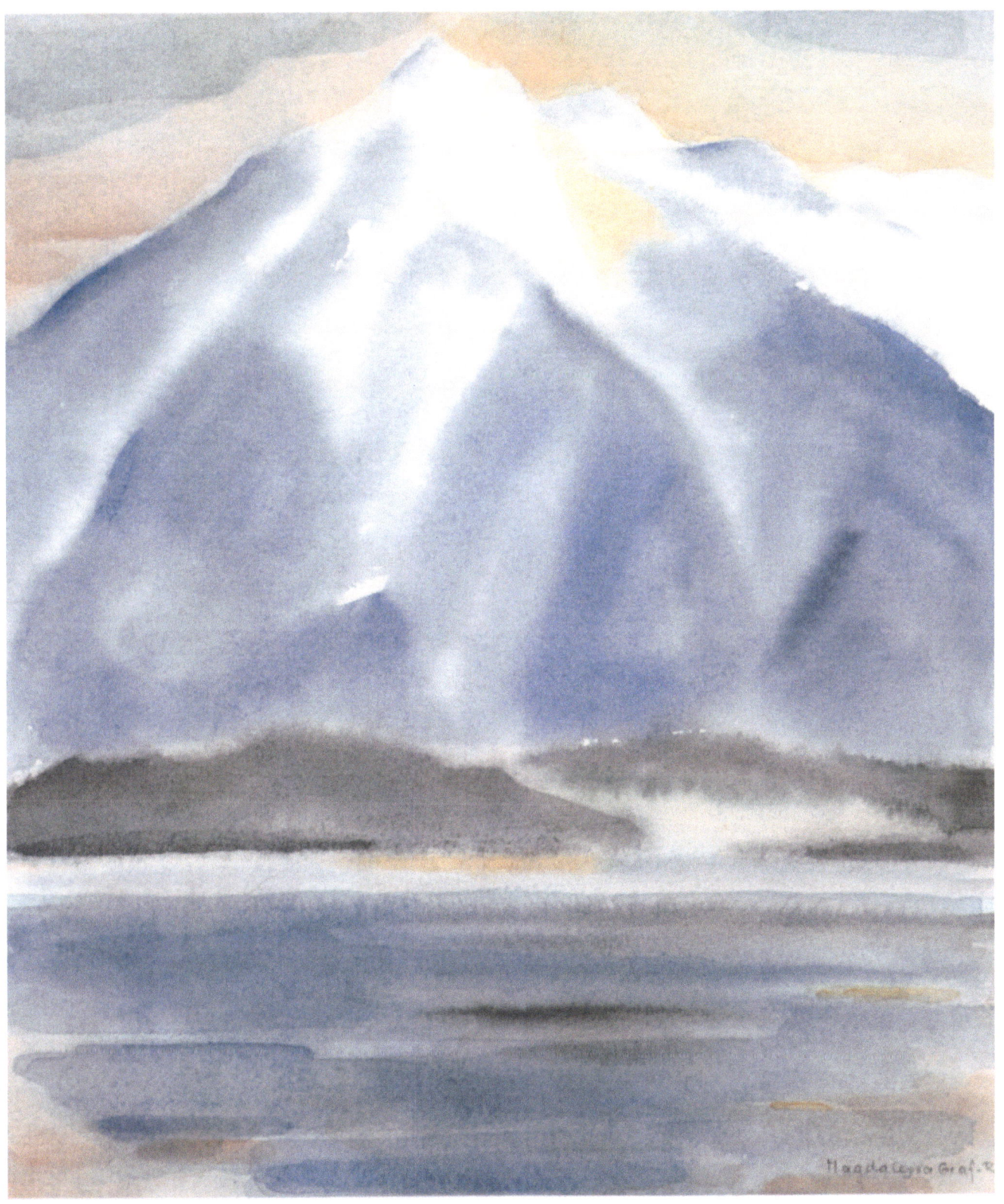

Alles, was ich sehe,
lehrt mich,
dem Schöpfer auch bei allem,
was ich nicht sehe,
zu vertrauen.

Whatever I see
makes me trust the Creator
even with everything
I cannot see

Ralph Waldo Emerson

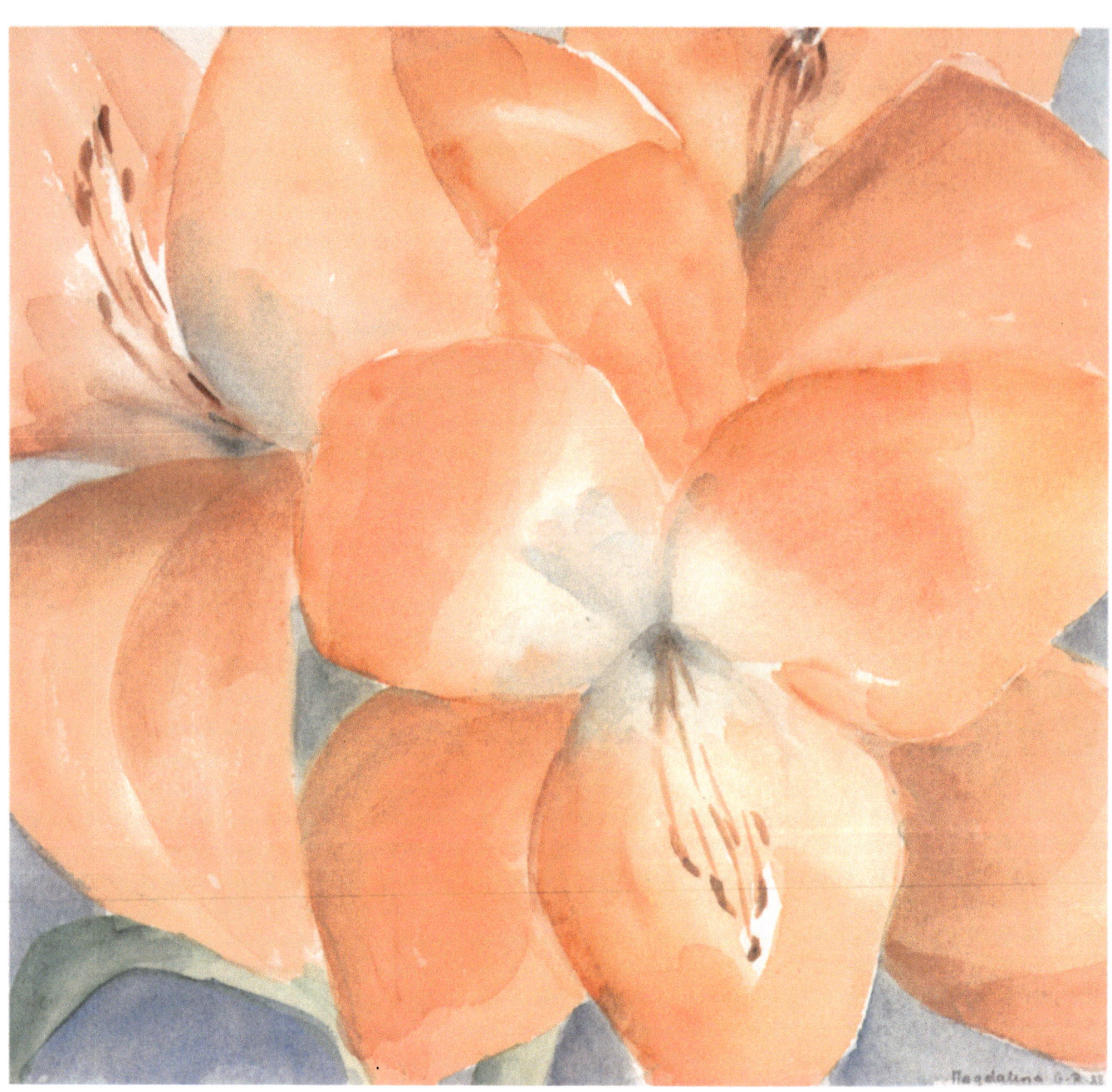

Magdalina G-R 88

in mir
singt ein lied
dank

in mir
singt ein lied
jubel

in mir
singt ein lied
freude

in mir
singt ein lied
gott

Josephine Hirsch

there is a song
in me
thanks

there is a song
in me
jubilation

there is a song
in me
joy

there is a song
in me
God

Danksagung

Zitate wurden mit freundlicher Genehmigung folgenden
Werken entnommen:

Marc Chagall, *Die großen Gemälde der Biblischen
Botschaft,* Belser, Stuttgart, 1986

Bernt von Heiseler, *Das verschwiegene Wort,* Stein-
kopf, Stuttgart, 1964, p. 239

Josephine Hirsch, *Träume,* Herold, Vienna, 1985

Acknowledgements

Citations were taken with permission from the following
sources:

Lawrence LeShan, *Psychotherapie gegen den Krebs,*
2. Aufl., aus dem Amerikanischen übersetzt von Si-
billa Marclli, Thomas Schadow und Ulrike Stopfel,
Klett-Cotta, Stuttgart, 1982, p. 192. Original Amer-
ican edition: *You Can Fight for Your Life.* Emotion-
al factors in the treatment of cancer. M. Evans &
Company, Inc., New York, 1977, p. 192